THE *Skinny*
gluten free
SLOW COOKER
RECIPE BOOK

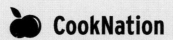

THE SKINNY GLUTEN FREE SLOW COOKER RECIPE BOOK
DELICIOUS GLUTEN FREE RECIPES UNDER 300, 400 AND 500 CALORIES

ISBN 978-1-911219-26-2

DISCLAIMER

Prepare the other ingredients for the rice salad following the recipe.

Discuss and then write out the conclusions you can draw from these experiments.

Which rice salad is better for your health? Explain your answer.

Investigate what other foods can be successfully cooked in the microwave oven (use recipe books to find this information). Compare the cooking times with those given for other methods of cooking.

Find out about the different types of microwave ovens available, including combination ovens. Find out the prices of different makes and models.

Evaluate your work.

Reading list and further sources of information:

The Electricity Council
30 Millbank, London SW19 4RD

The British Gas Education Service
PO Box 46, Hounslow, Middlesex TW4 6NF

Manufacturers of goods are generally pleased to supply information about their products and the Consumer Association test products and publish their findings in the 'Which Reports'.

The Consumers' Association
14 Buckingham Street, London WC2N 6DS

Computer software
Kitchen Planning in 3D

9 Safety and hygiene

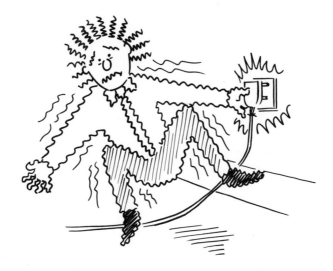

In an average year 1,000 people are killed in the workplace and over 500,000 are injured. These figures mean that every working day, four people are killed and 2,000 people are hurt, many of whom end up in hospital. Over 250,000 accidents occur in domestic kitchens each year, that represents nearly one in five of home accidents. Cuts, falls, burns, scalds and accidental poisonings are the main problems and many of the injuries are to children, but the whole family can be endangered if the hazards are not recognised.

Health and safety is an important issue today because of the large numbers of accidents that occur both at work and in the home. More people die from accidents at home than from accidents at work or anywhere else.

Health and safety at work

At people's places of work there will be a Health and Safety Officer. In schools there will be people responsible for health and safety.

1974 Health and Safety Act

In 1974 the Government passed a law called the Health and Safety Act. This stresses the need for each person to be aware of their responsibilities for the personal health and safety of themselves and others, so that firms, businesses and schools should make their work forces aware of safety rules and regulations.

CONTENTS

FISH & SEAFOOD

VEGETABLE/VEGETARIAN

DESSERTS 75

OTHER COOKNATION TITLES 91

You may also enjoy other Skinny Recipe Books by 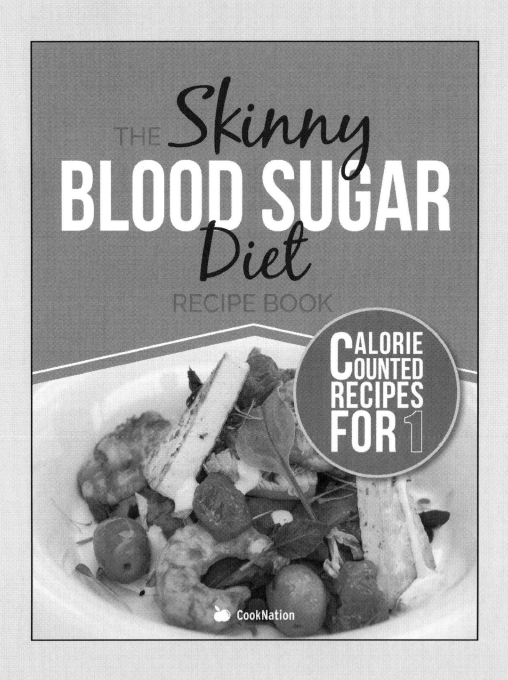 CookNation including:

THE *Skinny* BLOOD SUGAR *Diet* RECIPE BOOK

CALORIE COUNTED RECIPES FOR 1

CookNation

INTRODUCTION

Our skinny collection of recipes are perfect for those wishing to maintain a balanced, healthy, gluten free diet.

Slow cooking is an incredible method of preparing delicious meals. As well as being economical and convenient, the process of slow cooking ingredients to bring out the best in their flavour is unmatched.

For those who suffer from the effects of gluten in their diet and who love their slow cooker we have now created an appetizing collection of skinny gluten free recipes under 300, 400 and 500 calories that will help you make inexpensive, healthy meals for you and your family with the minimum of fuss.

Each recipe is free from gluten, uses simple and inexpensive fresh ingredients and packed full of flavour and goodness. Enjoy maximum taste with minimum calories without the effects that gluten causes in your diet.

One of the best things about a slow cooker is that it takes care of itself leaving you to attend to other things. What better appliance to have in the kitchen? The slow cooker can be your new best friend allowing you to enjoy free time, friends and family while the slow cooker does all the work.

Our skinny collection of recipes are perfect for those wishing to maintain a balanced, healthy, gluten free diet. Each recipe usually serves 4-6 people and all fall below either 300, 400 or 500 calories.

WHY GLUTEN FREE?

Gluten is a term for proteins found in wheat, rye, barley and any foods made with these grains. The presence of gluten causes significant issues to the health and wellbeing of many people. Your motive for going gluten free may fall under one of the following categories:

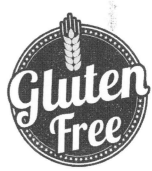

- Coeliac disease: an auto-immune condition where the effect of gluten in a diet damages the lining of the small intestine causing bloating, diarrhoea, nausea, tiredness and headaches.

- Gluten intolerance or sensitivity: experienced by many who do not have damage to the lining of their intestine however still experience symptoms such as headaches, bloating, fatigue, or diarrhea after eating foods that contain gluten.

  General healthy eating and weight management: many people now follow a gluten free diet as a means of creating a more nutritious and healthy lifestyle. By omitting gluten from meals, focus is placed more on a variety of whole foods such as vegetables, fruits, lean meats, seafood, dairy, and non-gluten grains like quinoa.

Whatever your driving force for following a gluten free diet, our skinny slow cooker recipes can help improve the quality of your life.

WHAT CAN I EAT?

Finding out which foods do and don't contain gluten can appear to be a minefield but the good news is there is a growing wealth of information freely available to coeliac sufferers and those with a gluten intolerance. We recommend visiting www. coeliac.org.uk who publish a monthly list of gluten free products.

There are too many foods to list that are gluten free (that's good news). Generally speaking wheat in all forms should be avoided e.g. barley & malt, rye, meat, fish and vegetables breaded in flour made from wheat. Meat, fish and vegetables with a marinade or sauce which contains gluten e.g. soy sauce. The exception to this is Buckwheat.

There are also many foods which neither fall into the 'gluten free' or 'contain gluten' categories which makes selecting ingredients more problematic. For example oats are considered gluten free however if these oats are processed in facilities that also process wheat, barley, and rye then cross contamination may occur.

All spices are gluten free however it is possible that some brands may use flour to prevent 'clumping'. This also applies to ingredients such as garlic, onion and chilli powders.

When in doubt we strongly recommend you read the label of each food product and if in doubt select a product labeled as gluten free. Throughout this recipe book we state when specific ingredients labeled as gluten free should be used.

COOKING THE SKINNY WAY WITH YOUR SLOW COOKER

Many of us can be guilty of overeating and making poor nutritional choices, which can often result in overeating, weight gain and sluggishness.

These delicious gluten free slow cooker recipes use simple, seasonal and inexpensive fresh and store-cupboard ingredients are packed full of flavour and goodness, and show that you can enjoy maximum taste with minimum calories.

Each recipe has been tried, tested, and enjoyed time and time again and we're sure you'll soon agree that diet can still mean delicious!

PREPARATION

Most of the recipes should take no longer than 10-15 minutes to prepare. Browning the meat will make a difference to the taste of your recipe, but if you really don't have the time, don't worry - it will still taste great.

All meat and vegetables should be cut into even sized pieces unless stated in the recipe. Some ingredients can take longer to cook than others, particularly root vegetables, but that has been allowed for in the cooking time. As much as possible meat should be trimmed of visible fat and the skin removed.

LOW COST

Slow cooking is ideal for cheaper meat cuts. The 'tougher' cuts used in this collection of recipes are transformed into meat which melts-in-your-mouth and helps to keep costs down. We've also made sure not to include one-off ingredients, which are used for a single recipe and never used again. All the herbs and spices listed can be used in multiple recipes throughout the book.

SLOW COOKER TIPS

All cooking times are a guide. Make sure you get to know your own slow cooker so that you can adjust timings accordingly.

Read the manufacturers operating instructions as appliances can vary. For example, some recommend preheating the slow cooker for 20 minutes before use whilst others advocate switching on only when you are ready to start cooking.

Slow cookers do not brown-off meat. While this is not always necessary, if you do prefer to brown your meat you must first do this in a pan with a little low calorie cooking spray.

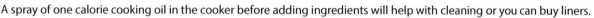

A spray of one calorie cooking oil in the cooker before adding ingredients will help with cleaning or you can buy liners.

Don't be tempted to regularly lift the lid of your appliance while cooking. The seal that is made with the lid on is all part of the slow cooking process. Each time you do lift the lid you will need to increase the cooking time.

Removing the lid at the end of the cooking time can be useful to thicken up a sauce by adding additional cooking time and continuing to cook without the lid on. On the other hand if perhaps a sauce it too thick removing the lid and adding a little more liquid can help.

Always add hot liquids to your slow cooker, not cold.

Do not overfill your slow cooker.

Allow the inner dish of your slow cooker to completely cool before cleaning. Any stubborn marks can usually be removed after a period of soaking in hot soapy water.

Be confident with your cooking. Feel free to use substitutes to suit your own taste and don't let a missing herb or spice stop you making a meal - you'll almost always be able to find something to replace it.

OUR RECIPES

The recipes in this book are all low calorie, gluten free dishes mainly serving 4-6, which make it easier for you to monitor your overall daily calorie intake as well as those you are cooking for. The recommended daily calories are approximately 2000 for women and 2500 for men.

Broadly speaking, by consuming the recommended levels of calories each day you should maintain your current weight. Reducing the number of calories (a calorie deficit) will result in losing weight. This happens because the body begins to use fat stores for energy to make up the reduction in calories, which in turn results in weight loss. We have already counted the calories for each dish making it easy for you to fit this into your daily eating plan whether you want to lose weight, maintain your current figure or are just looking for some great-tasting, skinny slow cooker meals.

I'M ALREADY ON A DIET. CAN I USE THESE RECIPES?

Yes of course. All the recipes can be great accompaniments to many of the popular calorie-counting diets. We all know that sometimes dieting can result in hunger pangs, cravings and boredom from eating the same old foods day in and day out. Our skinny slow cooker recipes provide filling meals that should satisfy you for hours afterwards.
I Am Only Cooking For One. Will This Book Work For Me?
Yes. We would recommend following the method for the stated number of servings then dividing and storing the rest in single size portions for you to use in the future. Most of the recipes will freeze well. Allow your slow cooked meals to cool to room temperature before refrigerating or freezing. When ready to defrost, allow to thaw in a fridge overnight then at room temperature for a few hours depending on the size of portion. Reheat thoroughly.

NUTRITION

All of the recipes in this collection are balanced low calorie meals that should keep you feeling full and help you avoid snacking in-between meals.
If you are following a diet, it is important to balance your food between proteins, good carbs, dairy, fruit and vegetables.

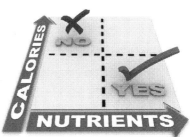

Protein. Keeps you feeling full and is also essential for building body tissue. Good protein sources come from meat, fish and eggs.

Carbohydrates. Carbs are generally high in calories, which make them difficult to include in a calorie limiting diet. Carbs are a good source of energy for your body as they are converted more easily into glucose (sugar), providing energy. Try to eat 'good carbs' which are high in fibre and nutrients e.g. whole fruits and veg, nuts, seeds, whole grain cereals, beans and legumes.

Dairy. Dairy products provide you with vitamins and minerals. Cheeses can be high in calories but other products such as fat free Greek yoghurt, crème fraiche and skimmed milk are all good.

Fruit & Vegetables. Eat your five a day. There is never a better time to fill your 5 a day quota. Not only are fruit and veg very healthy, they also fill up your plate and are ideal snacks when you are feeling hungry.

We have adopted theses broader nutritional principals in all our recipes.

PORTION SIZES

The majority of recipes are for 4-6 servings servings. The calorie count is based on one serving. It is important to remember that if you are aiming to lose weight using any of our skinny recipes, the size of the portion that you put on your plate will significantly affect your weight loss efforts. Filling your plate with over-sized portions will obviously increase your calorie intake and hamper your dieting efforts.
It is important with all meals that you use a correct sized portion, which generally is the size of your clenched fist.
This applies to any side dishes of vegetables and carbs too.

ALL RECIPES ARE A GUIDE ONLY

All the recipes in this book are a guide only. You may need to alter quantities and cooking times to suit your own appliances.

ABOUT COOKNATION

CookNation is the leading publisher of innovative and practical recipe books for the modern, health conscious cook.

CookNation titles bring together delicious, easy and practical recipes with their unique approach - easy and delicious, no-nonsense recipes - making cooking for diets and healthy eating fast, simple and fun.

With a range of #1 best-selling titles - from the innovative 'Skinny' calorie-counted series, to the 5:2 Diet Recipes collection - CookNation recipe books prove that 'Diet' can still mean 'Delicious'!

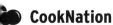 **CookNation**

THE *Skinny* *gluten free* SLOW COOKER

RECIPE BOOK

Meat & Poultry

CUBAN STEW

453 calories per serving

Ingredients

- 550g/1¼lb lean braising steak
- Salt & black pepper to taste
- ½ medium onion, peeled & chopped
- 60g/2½oz gluten free salsa
- 1 green chilli, seeded & chopped
- 1 tomato, chopped
- 1 tsp garlic powder

- 1 red pepper, seeded & cut into strips
- 1 yellow pepper, seeded & cut into strips
- 1 tbsp ground cumin
- ½ tbsp ground coriander
- ½ tsp dried oregano
- ½ tbsp chilli powder
- 1 tbsp apple cider vinegar

Method

1 Season the meat with salt and pepper and sear it a hot pan until browned on all sides. Place the meat in the bottom of the slow cooker.

2 Add the onion, salsa, chillies, and tomatoes to the pan you seared the meat in. Stir to scrape up any browned meat, and bring to a boil. Pour it over the meat in the slow cooker.

3 Add the rest of the ingredients and combine well.

4 Cook for at least 4 hours on High, or 6 hours on Low, or until the meat is tender and cooked through.

CHEFS NOTE

Some salsa contains vinegar, which may have been distilled from glutinous grains, so if you don't make your own salsa verde, take care which you buy.

PULLED PORK WITH WHISKY

412 calories per serving

Ingredients

- ½ tbsp olive oil
- 2 tsp smoked paprika
- 1 tsp salt
- 1 tsp freshly ground black pepper
- 1½kg/3lb 6oz pork shoulder roast (with bone in)
- 120ml/½ cup gluten free hot chicken stock
- 4 tbsp balsamic vinegar
- 4 tbsp black treacle
- 2 tbsp gluten free soy sauce
- 1 tsp crushed chilli
- 175g/6oz peach preserve or jam
- 2 onions, peeled & thinly sliced
- 5 garlic cloves, peeled & thinly sliced
- 60ml/¼ cup whisky
- 2 tbsp cold water
- 2 tsp cornflour

Method

Heat the oil in a large pan over a medium-high heat. In a small bowl combine the paprika, half the salt, and all the pepper. Rub the mixture evenly over the pork and brown it evenly in the pan for around 10 minutes.

Place the pork in the slow cooker. Add the stock, vinegar, treacle, soy sauce and crushed chilli to the browning pan and bring to a boil, scraping the pan to loosen browned bits. Add the peach preserve and whisk.

Pour the mixture over the pork in the slow cooker. Add the onion and garlic. Cover and cook on Low for 5-6½ hours or until the pork is very tender.

Remove the pork, cool slightly, then shred the meat with 2 forks. Remove the onion from the slow cooker with a slotted spoon and add it to the pork.

5 Pour the liquid from the slow cooker into a bowl, leave to cool a bit and skim off the fat. Pour the liquid into a small pan with the whisky and bring to the boil. Cook for about 10 minutes to reduce the liquid.

6 Combine the cold water and cornflour in a small bowl, whisking into a smooth paste. Add it to the pan, stirring constantly until the sauce thickens. Pour it over the pork, and serve.

CHEFS NOTE

Use red wine instead of whisky if you prefer.

CHICKEN, BACON AND BEER

410 calories per serving

Ingredients

- 5 rashers back bacon
- 3 tbsp all-purpose gluten-free flour
- 1kg/2¼lb boneless, skinless chicken thighs
- 370ml/1½ cups gluten-free beer
- 120ml/½ cup gluten free hot chicken stock
- 2 tbsp barbecue sauce

- 1 tsp dried oregano
- ½ tsp dried thyme
- ¼ tsp sea salt
- ¼ tsp freshly ground pepper
- 1 tbsp water
- 2 tsp tapioca or arrowroot starch

Method

1 Cook the bacon under the grill until crispy. Leave to cool and chop finely.

2 Toss the chicken thighs in the flour until coated, then place in the bottom of the slow cooker.

3 In a bowl, mix together the bacon pieces, beer, stock, barbecue sauce and herbs. Then pour the mixture over the chicken in the slow cooker. Cover and cook on Low for 8-9 hours or High for 4-5 hours. Ensure the chicken it cooked through.

4 Combine the water and starch in a small bowl to make a smooth paste. Set aside.

5 Remove the chicken with a slotted spoon and place in a bowl. Cover with foil to keep warm.

6 Stir the starch mixture in with leftover chicken liquids in the slow cooker. Whisk until combined. Cover and cook, on Low, for 15 minutes to make a 'gravy'.

7 Drizzle the gravy over the chicken and serve.

CHEFS NOTE
Like gluten free flour, you can now buy gluten free beer from most large supermarkets.

SATSUMA CHICKEN

394 calories per serving

Ingredients

- 6 skin-on chicken thighs
- 2 tsp Chinese Five Spice
- ½ tsp salt
- 225g/8oz satsuma slices
- 2 garlic cloves, crushed
- 1 tbsp grated ginger

- ½ red chilli, seeded & finely chopped
- 1 tbsp lime juice
- 1 tbsp brown sugar
- 1 tsp sesame oil
- 2 tbsp fish sauce

Method

1 Rub the chicken thighs with the five spice powder and salt.

2 In a hot frying pan, sear the chicken for about 3 minutes on each side.

3 Lay the chicken in the slow cooker, skin side up. Combine the rest of the ingredients in a small bowl and mix well. Pour this over the chicken in the slow cooker.

4 Cook on High for 4 hours, or Low for 6 hours. Check the chicken is tender and cooked through, and then remove to a serving dish.

5 Use a hand blender to puree the sauce in the bottom of the slow cooker, or spoon it into a blender.

6 Whizz until the sauce is smooth then pour it over the chicken. Serve warm.

CHEFS NOTE
For convenience, use tinned mandarin oranges (with no added sugar) instead of fresh satsumas if you wish.

BEEF CURRY

350
calories per
serving

Ingredients

- 500g/1lb 2oz lean braising steak
- 4 tbsp coconut milk powder
- 250ml/1 cup water
- 2 tbsp red curry paste
- 3 cardamom pods, cracked
- 1 tbsp fish sauce
- 1 tsp onion powder
- 1 red chilli, seeded & chopped

- ½ tbsp ground cumin
- ½ tbsp ground coriander
- ½ tsp ground cloves
- ½ tsp ground nutmeg
- ½ tbsp ground ginger
- ½ tbsp granulated sweetener
- 75g/3oz cashews, roughly chopped
- 2 tsp freshly chopped coriander, chopped

Method

1 Place the meat in the slow cooker. Add 3 tbsp coconut milk powder, water, 1½ tbsp red curry paste, fish sauce, cardamom pods, onion flakes, chillies, cumin, ground coriander, cloves, nutmeg, and ginger.

2 Cover and cook on High for about 5 hours, or on Low for 8 hours. Just before serving, remove the meat to another dish. Whisk into the liquid the remaining 1 tbsp coconut milk powder, and ½ tbsp curry paste.

3 Shred or chop the meat into smaller pieces. Stir it into the sauce, along with the chopped cashews.

4 Serve garnished with fresh chopped coriander.

CHEFS NOTE
Delicious with coconut and lime flavoured cauliflower rice.

One such firm BP, issue a booklet to all their staff.

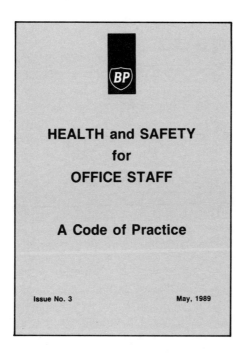

The staff are required to read the instructions carefully and comply with the relevant sections whilst they are at work, e.g.

Section 1   Applicable to all staff.
Section 2   Applicable to special computer areas, and the staff who work in them.
Section 3   Applicable to other areas with machinery or specialised equipment and the staff who work in them.

School is your place of work and different areas will have health and safety officers responsible for it.

Health and safety in the home

In the home one area where there are many hazards is the kitchen. Inevitably many accidents occur here.

 Investigation

Level 1
Draw a plan of your own kitchen at home. Indicate safety features with a green dot and unsafe areas with a red dot. How can you make the unsafe areas safe?

As well as the kitchen at home, safety rules apply to the Home Economics rooms in school.

Investigation

Level 1

Investigate the health and safety rules that apply to activities in the classroom. Ask your teacher if you could observe a practical lesson in another class. Write down the health and safety rules for the room that you feel are necessary from your observations.

Accidents also happen:

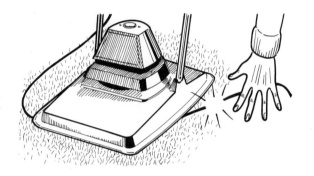

In the garden

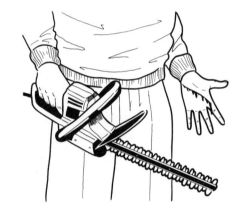

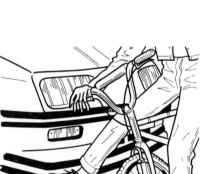

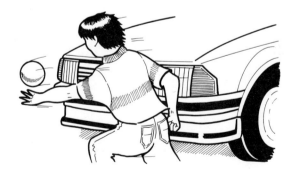

On the road

1 What safety rules should be followed when using garden equipment?
2 Think of ten other rules that should be observed for garden safety.

Compare your answers with the other members of the class.

Safety on the roads is important for children and adults. Legislation has been passed by the Government to make the wearing of seat belts compulsory because of the number of drivers and passengers who were badly injured or killed by going through the car's windscreen.

Worksheet

Now try and answer the questions on Worksheets 32 and 33, you can check your answers on Worksheet 34 and then look at Worksheet 35 and 36.

Hygiene in the kitchen

The kitchen should be kept very clean. The surfaces, cooking utensils, knives and any equipment that comes into contact with food and the food itself have the potential of being **dangerous**.

There are **micro-organisms** in the air that can contaminate food; these are yeasts, moulds and bacteria. Some of these micro-organisms are harmful and can cause **food poisoning**.

Three more cases of food poisoning

Three young girls aged 16 and 17 have been rushed to hospital after having eaten in a West End restaurant. It is suspected that they are suffering from salmonella food poisoning caused by chicken. Sarah Taylor, Linda Rowlands and Alison Harvie are all said to be in a stable condition.

Beware

An outbreak of food poisoning seems to have come from food that has been re-heated in microwave cookers. A spokesperson stressed that food must always be thoroughly re-heated.

Old people at risk

At Newbridge Old People's Home, four residents have been diagnosed as having food poisoning. This is believed to have come from tinned fish. They will be kept in hospital for five days.

Causes of food contamination

Do you know any more?

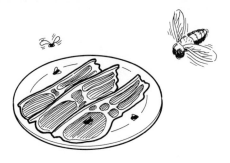

Flies on food

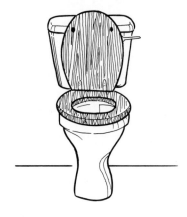

Not washing hands

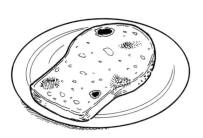

Food uncovered

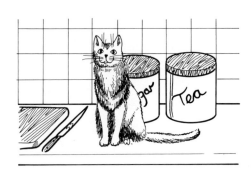

Pets in the kitchen

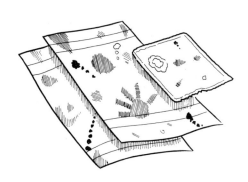

Dirty dishcloths and teatowels

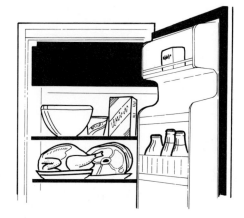

Cooked and raw meat stored together

The ideal conditions for the growth of such micro-organisms are in warm temperatures, on food and on moisture.

Safe uses of micro-organisms

Some of these micro-organisms are useful, for example yeast is required in bread-making and moulds are used in blue cheeses.

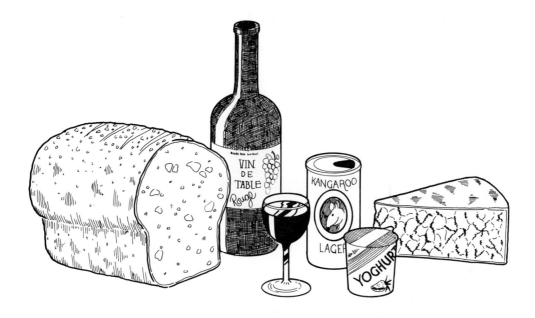

Harmful effects of micro-organisms

However, certain micro-organisms can cause food to go bad and given the right conditions for growth can contaminate the food, which can cause it to become **toxic** and lead to food poisoning.

Food will go rotten because of the **chemical enzymes** in it. These speed up the breakdown of the cell walls of the food causing them to become soft and discoloured. An immediate result of enzyme action can be seen when preparing some fruits and vegetables. They quickly go brown.

 Investigation

Level 2
Investigate the action of enzymes in one of the following foods:

apples
bananas
potatoes.

Carry out experiments to find ways of preventing this enzyme action.

In the experiments investigate the effect of alkali, acid, heat and water on these foods.

Investigation

Level 1

Devise a game for use with first year pupils to help them understand and remember the concept of safety or hygiene in the home. You may need some of the following pieces of equipment and materials:

Coloured card
Coloured paper
Gummed paper
Scissors
Glue
Sellotape
Felt pens
Pencil
Ruler
Crayons
Tacky-back adhesive sheets
Stencils

For a sensible evaluation of the games use them with first year classes. Devise a questionnaire for them to give their opinions on the usefulness of the games.

Level 1/2/3

Arrange a visit to one of the following:

A local firm,
A hospital,
Your school kitchen,
A local supermarket.

Assess the health, safety and hygiene practices within this establishment.

Find out who is responsible for health, safety and hygiene in the establishment of your choice.

Interview this person if it is possible, asking some of the following questions:

1 What rules apply regarding health, safety and hygiene?
2 Are there different rules for different parts of the building?
3 What are the most common accidents and how are these being prevented?
4 Where are exit points/fire stations/fire extinguishers in case of fire?

You may find other questions to ask on your visit from things you see. Do you think safety and hygiene standards are being met according to the 1974 Act?

Reading list and further sources of information:

ROSPA
Kitchen Safety Campaign *(kitchen safety resource pack)*
Common House, The Priory, Queensway, Birmingham B4 6BS

Danger Men at Work
IEHO
Clive Wadey, Assistant Secretary
or Kim Fricker, Education Liaison Officer (Tel: 01 928 0606)

Video
Hygiene in Action
Domestos Advisory Service
50 Upper Brook Street, London W1Y 1PG
(leaflets and fact sheets also available)

10 Know your rights

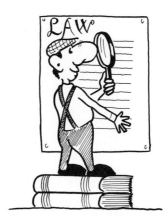

When the consumer buys something a contract is made between them and the seller. The seller is obliged by law to sort out a complaint. This law is called **The 1979 Sale of Goods Act**.

It has three rules. These are that:

1 The goods should be of a merchantable quality. This means that they should not be broken or damaged. They should not be faulty.
2 The goods should be what they say they are. If an item says 'leather handbag' then it should not be plastic.
3 The goods should be 'fit for the purpose intended'. In other words, if a casserole dish is described as resistant to heat, then it should be.

This act covers all goods bought from shops, street traders, door to door salesmen and catalogues. It includes food and sale items.

What do you do if you buy something that does not work?

You must tell the seller immediately. If any of the three rules are broken then you can:
- have a money refund or
- have a replacement item or free repair or
- get a cash payment that is the difference between the original cost and the reduced value.

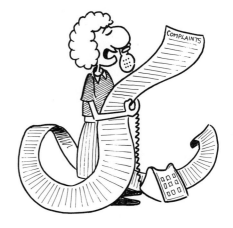

Making a complaint

When you find you have a faulty item:

1 Do not continue to use it.
2 Inform the shop or supplier.
3 Return the item to the shop or supplier if it is possible.
4 Keep a receipt.
5 Ask for the assistant who served you if this is possible or the manager.
6 Be clear about what has happened and what you want.

Complaining by letter

1 Always use recorded delivery.
2 Keep a copy of the letter.
3 Do not send guarantees or receipts.
  Send photocopies or give reference numbers.

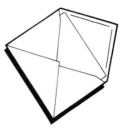

You have had a new food processor for two weeks. It has developed a fault. Write a letter to explain the fault and state what compensation you expect.

Complaining by phone

1 Make sure you know what to say.
2 Know who you are speaking to and keep a record of that person's name.
3 Have all the information you need to hand.

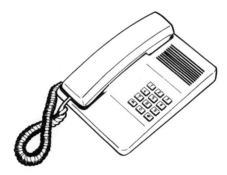

Guarantees

Manufacturers of goods often offer a guarantee. This can also protect the consumer. If the guarantee runs out still make the complaint. A guarantee cannot be limited to a particular time span. The manufacturer is liable at all times if goods are defective.

Role play

In groups of two or three imagine you are in a situation where you have to re-enact returning faulty goods to a shop. Think of a situation you may know about or make one up.

As a last resort, if you are unable to get satisfaction you can contact **The Office of Fair Trading** and **The Citizen's Advice Bureau** who will offer help.

Investigation

Level 2

Certain goods are tested before they are put on the market. Devise a series of tests for oven gloves which you consider would make them safe.

Are there any you consider to be unsafe and yet are still on sale?

Tabulate your results.

What is meant by the kitemark?

Reading list and further sources of information:

Which Reports
The Consumers Association
14 Buckingham Street, London WC2N 6DS

Local Citizens Advice Bureau (CAB)
Telephone number in Yellow Pages

The Office of Fair Trading
Field House, 15–25 Breams Buildings, London EC4A 1PR

Advertising Standards Authority
2–16 Torrington Place, London WE1 7NH

British Standards Institution (BSI)
2 Park Street, London W1A 2BS

COURGETTE AND MEAT LOAF

358 calories per serving

Ingredients

- 900g/2lb lean steak mince
- 2 large eggs
- 1 medium courgette, shredded
- 50g/2oz Parmesan cheese, grated
- 1 tbsp flat leaf parsley, finely chopped
- 4 cloves garlic, crushed
- 3 tbsp balsamic vinegar
- 1 tbsp dried oregano
- 1 tbsp onion powder

- ½ tsp salt
- ½ tsp freshly ground black pepper
- Coconut oil spray
- For Topping:
- 50g/2oz gluten free ketchup
- 50g/2oz low fat grated Mozzarella cheese
- 1 tbsp flat leaf parsley, finely chopped

Method

1. In a large bowl, combine all the ingredients (except those for the topping) and combine well.

2. Line the bottom of the slow cooker with aluminium foil, lengthwise and breadthwise, leaving flaps that will enable you to easily lift out the meatloaf once it's ready. Spray the bottom with coconut oil.

3. Place the mixture in the slow cooker and shape it into a meatloaf with your hands. Cover and cook on Low for 5-6 hours or on High for 3-4 hours.

4. Spread ketchup on top of the meatloaf and sprinkle with cheese. Cover and cook for another 5 minutes, or until cheese is melted. Remove the meatloaf from the slow cooker, and sprinkle with parsley.

CHEFS NOTE
The meatloaf can be refrigerated for up to 3 days, or frozen in an airtight container for up to a month.

19

CHICKEN ENCHILADAS

490 calories per serving

Ingredients

- 1 tsp olive oil
- 1 medium onion, peeled & chopped
- 1 red chilli seeded & chopped
- 2 cloves garlic, crushed
- 1 tsp chilli powder
- 400g/14oz tin chopped tomatoes, drained
- 225g/8oz tin tomato passata/sieved tomatoes
- 1 tsp dried mixed herbs

- Cooking spray
- 250g/9oz chicken breast, cooked & shredded
- 175g/6oz sweetcorn
- 400g/14oz tin black beans, rinsed & drained
- 5 gluten free soft tortillas
- 225g/8oz reduced-fat mature Cheddar cheese, grated
- Coriander sprigs, to garnish

Method

1 Heat the olive oil in a large pan over medium-high heat. Add the onion, chopped chilli & garlic and gently sauté for a few minutes.

2 Stir in the chilli powder, tomatoes and passata.

3 Coat the slow cooker with cooking spray. Spread 3 tbsp of the tomato mixture from the pan onto the bottom of the slow cooker. Combine the remaining tomato mixture with the chicken, corn, and beans.

4 Place one tortilla on top of the sauce in slow cooker. Layer on the chicken mixture, some cheese, another tortilla and so on, finishing with cheese.

5 Cover and cook on Low for 2 hours or until the cheese melts and the edges are lightly browned.

6 Garnish with the coriander sprigs, and cut into 8 wedges.

CHEFS NOTE
Adjust the chilli to suit your own taste.

EASY SAUSAGE AND BEAN CASSEROLE

357 calories per serving

Ingredients

- 8 gluten free sausages
- 2 x 400g/14oz tins mixed beans
- 2 x 400g/14oz tins chopped tomato
- 1 tsp dried basil
- 2 tsp dried oregano
- 1 tbsp sugar
- Salt and pepper

Method

1 Brown the sausages in a non-stick frying pan over a high heat for 3-5 minutes. Transfer them to the slow cooker and add the beans.

2 Add one tin of tomatoes to the slow cooker. Drain the other tin and pour the tomatoes without the juice into the slow cooker. Stir in the herbs and sugar cover and cook on Low for up to 6-8 hours or until the sausages are cooked through and piping hot.

CHEFS NOTE
Adding a little sugar brings out the natural sweetness of tomatoes.

SPICED PORK RIBS

415 calories per serving

Ingredients

- 1½kg/3lb 6oz pork ribs
- 250ml/1 cup gluten free barbecue sauce (use only half in the slow cooker)
- 2 gluten free stock cubes
- 2 bay leaves

- 1 tsp coriander seeds
- 1 tsp mustard seeds
- 1 tsp peppercorns
- 1½lt/6 cups water

Method

1 Add all the ingredients to the slow cooker (using only half the barbecue sauce). Top up with enough water to cover the ribs (around 1½lt). Cook on Low for around 8 hours until the meat is very tender but not completely falling off the bone.

2 Heat the oven to 220C/200C Fan. Carefully remove the ribs from the slow cooker using a slotted spoon or tongs. Baste them with the remaining barbecue sauce and lay them on a foil-lined baking tray. Cook for 20–30 minutes until starting to crisp.

CHEFS NOTE

You can cook the ribs in the slow cooker the day before, baste them in barbecue sauce, cover and refrigerate overnight before either oven-cooking or barbecuing them.

COCONUT BEEF CURRY

497
calories per serving

Ingredients

- 1 tbsp peanut oil
- 900g/2lb beef brisket, cut into large chunks
- 25g/1oz coriander
- 1 stalk lemongrass, roughly chopped
- 2 cloves garlic, peeled & chopped
- 1 small green chilli, seeded & chopped
- 1 tsp fresh grated ginger
- 1 tbsp rice wine vinegar
- 1 tbsp fish sauce
- 1 tbsp brown sugar
- 250ml/1 cup light coconut milk
- 1 star anise
- 3 kaffir lime leaves
- 1 tbsp lime juice

Method

1 Switch the slow cooker on to High.

2 Heat a little of the oil in a large pan and brown the beef.

3 Combine half the coriander, the lemongrass, garlic and chillies with the rest of the oil until you have a rough paste.

4 Heat the paste in the pan for a few minutes, then add the beef and all the remaining ingredients (apart from the left over coriander and lime juice).

5 Turn the slow cooker down to Low and cook for 8 hrs, or until the meat is very tender. Stir in the remaining coriander and lime juice, then season with more fish sauce.

CHEFS NOTE
If you like, use beef ribs instead of brisket, and pull the meat from the bone after cooking.

SPICY CHICKEN AND TOMATO STEW

204 calories per serving

Ingredients

- 1 tbsp vegetable oil
- 1 medium onion, finely chopped
- 3 cloves garlic, crushed
- ½ tsp brown sugar
- 1 tsp chilli paste

- 400g/14oz tin chopped tomatoes
- 500g/1lb skinless chicken breasts
- 1 red onion, sliced into rings
- 1 tbsp chopped coriander leaves

Method

1 Heat the oil in a medium saucepan. Add the onion & garlic and gently sauté for 5 minutes until softened.

2 Add to the slow cooker and stir in the sugar, chilli paste, tomatoes and chicken. Cover and cook on High for 2 hours-3 hours or until the chicken is cooked through.

3 Remove the chicken and shred with 2 forks, then stir back into the sauce. Scatter with the red onion rings and coriander.

CHEFS NOTE
Serve with rice, or with corn tortillas.

VEGETABLES AND CHICKEN

340 calories per serving

Ingredients

- 500g/1lb skin-on chicken breasts
- 2 tbsp olive oil
- 2 medium potatoes, peeled and thinly sliced
- 1lt/4 cups gluten free hot chicken stock
- 400g/14oz mixed spring vegetables e.g. broccoli, peas, broad beans
- 4 tbsp crème fraîche
- A few tarragon leaves, roughly chopped

Method

1 Brown the chicken, skin-side down in a frying pan for 5 minutes. Turn the chicken over then stir in the potatoes for another minute.

2 Spread the potatoes along the bottom of the slow cooker. Lay the chicken breasts on top. Pour over half the stock, then cover and cook on High for an hour and a half.

3 Remove the chicken and stir in the vegetables. Put the chicken back on top and cook for another hour or until the chicken is cooked through and the vegetables are tender.

4 Stir in the crème fraîche to make a creamy sauce, season with salt and pepper.

5 Sprinkle with tarragon and serve.

CHEFS NOTE
Vary the green vegetables according to the season.

BOLOGNESE

355
calories per
serving

Ingredients

- 2 tbsp olive oil
- 3 rashers smoked back bacon, chopped
- 750g/1lb 11oz lean minced beef
- 2 onions, peeled & finely chopped
- 1 large carrot, peeled & finely chopped
- 2 stalks celery, finely chopped
- 250g/9oz mushrooms, sliced
- 4 cloves garlic, crushed

- 1 tbsp dried mixed herbs
- 1 bay leaf
- 3 x 400g/14oz tins chopped tomatoes
- 2 tbsp tomato purée/paste
- 2 tbsp red wine vinegar
- ½ tbsp sugar
- Salt and pepper

Method

1 Heat the oil in a large frying pan. Fry the bacon and brown the mince, then tip it all into the slow cooker. Add the vegetables, garlic, herbs, tomatoes, tomato purée, wine, vinegar, sugar and seasoning.

2 Cover and cook on Low for 6-8 hours, then uncover, turn up to High and cook for another hour until thick.

CHEFS NOTE
Serve with gluten free spaghetti and grated parmesan.

PORK AND PLUM CASSEROLE

496 calories per serving

Ingredients

- 750g/1lb 11oz pork shoulder
- 2 tbsp rice wine
- 3 tbsp gluten free soy sauce
- 1 tsp grated root ginger
- 3 cloves garlic, crushed
- ½ red chilli, seeded & finely chopped
- 1 tbsp vegetable oil
- 3 spring onions, finely sliced

- 1 star anise
- 1 tsp five-spice powder
- 1 cinnamon stick
- 1 tbsp sugar
- 1 tbsp tomato purée
- 250ml/1 cup gluten free hot chicken stock
- 4 ripe plums, stoned & chopped

Method

1 Cut the pork into approximately 4cm/2-inch cubes. Place in a bowl and add the wine, soy sauce, half the ginger, half the garlic and half the chilli. Marinate for at least 1 hour, or up to 24 hours.

2 Heat the vegetable oil in a large pan gently sauté the spring onions, the remaining ginger, garlic, chilli, cinnamon, star anise, five-spice, sugar and tomato purée. When the onions are soft remove to a plate. Increase the heat add the pork, and quickly fry each side until sealed.

3 Tip everything into the slow cooker. Cover and cook on Low for 8-9 hours. Skim off any surface fat and about an hour before the end of cooking, stir in the plums.

4 Scatter the remaining spring onions over the top, and serve.

CHEFS NOTE

The pork should be super-tender after this extended period of slow cooking.

BACON AND CHICKEN STEW

325 calories per serving

Ingredients

- 1 tbsp olive oil
- 6 chicken thighs, skinless
- 12 rashers smoked streaky bacon, chopped
- 200g/7oz shallots, peeled & chopped
- 2 medium potatoes, peeled & quartered
- A few sprigs thyme
- 250ml/1 cup gluten free white wine
- 500ml/2 cups hot chicken stock
- Squeeze of lemon juice
- 2 tbsp tarragon, chopped
- Salt and pepper

Method

1 Heat the oil in a large saucepan on a high heat and brown the chicken thighs for about 10 minutes, until they are golden. Remove them and set aside. Reduce the heat, add the bacon and shallots to the pan and gently sauté for a few minutes.

2 Add everything to the slow cooker, except the lemon juice and 1 tbsp tarragon. Cover and cook on High for 4-6 hours or until the chicken is really tender and falling off the bone.

3 Sprinkle in the lemon juice and remaining tarragon. Season with salt and pepper, and serve.

CHEFS NOTE
If you prefer not to use alcohol, this recipe is still tasty without the wine!

MOROCCAN LAMB SHANKS

496 calories per serving

Ingredients

- 3 tsp extra-virgin olive oil
- 1¼kg/2¾lb lamb shanks
- 1 large onion, chopped
- 2 cloves garlic, crushed
- 1¼ tsp sea salt
- 1 tsp saffron threads
- ¾ tsp cinnamon
- ½ tsp cayenne pepper
- 500ml/2 cups water
- 400g/14oz tin chopped tomatoes
- 400g/14oz tin chickpeas, drained
- 1 tbsp honey
- 1 tbsp chopped flat leaf parsley

Method

1 Heat 1 tsp oil in a large pan over medium heat. Add the lamb shanks to the pan and brown on all sides for a minute or two. Put the lamb to one side.

2 Add the remaining oil to the pan and gently sauté the onion, garlic and salt for a few minutes until softened. Stir in the saffron, cinnamon and cayenne pepper. Add water and bring to the boil.

3 Add everything to the slow cooker. Cover and cook on Low for 6-7 hours or until the lamb is cooked through and tender.

4 At the end of cooking you can shred the lamb off the bone and then stir back into the stew before serving.

CHEFS NOTE
Serve with rice or salad and lemon wedges.

CHICKEN, HAM AND BEAN STEW

298 calories per serving

Ingredients

- 1 onion, chopped
- 225g/8oz haricot beans, rinsed
- 225g/8oz boneless, skinless chicken thighs, cubed
- 175g/6oz ham, cubed
- 1 tsp dried mixed herbs
- ½ tsp ground black pepper

- ¼ tsp nutmeg
- 1lt/4 cups gluten free hot chicken stock
- 150g/5oz kale, roughly chopped
- 1 tbsp fresh sage, chopped
- 3 tsp lemon juice
- ½ tsp salt
- 1 tbsp chopped flat leaf parsley

Method

1 Add the onions, beans, chicken, ham, dried herbs, pepper and nutmeg into the slow cooker. Pour in the stock, combine well, cover and cook on Low for 7-8 hours.

2 When there is about an hour of cooking time remaining, stir in the kale, sage, lemon juice and salt. Cover and leave to finish cooking. Garnish with parsley before serving.

CHEFS NOTE
Use spinach or spring greens in the place of kale if you wish.

SWEET AND SPICY RIBS

499 calories per serving

Ingredients

- 800g/1¾lb beef ribs
- 1 tsp salt
- 1 tbsp canola oil + 1 tsp
- 450g/1lb mushrooms, sliced
- 2 tbsp brown sugar

- 2 tbsp gluten free soy sauce
- 2 tsp finely grated ginger root
- 1 tsp toasted sesame oil
- Pinch red chilli flakes

Method

1 Sprinkle the ribs with salt. Heat 1 tbsp oil in a large pan over high heat, and brown the ribs on both sides. Then place them bone-side down in your slow cooker.

2 Add the remaining tsp oil to the pan and reduce the heat. Add the mushrooms and sauté for a few minutes. Remove them from heat and stir in the sugar, soy sauce, ginger, sesame oil and red chilli flakes.

3 Pour the mushroom mixture over the ribs. Cover and cook on Low for 6 hours.

4 Take out the ribs using tongs, and divide them between 4 plates. Spoon the fat off the surface of the sauce, then pour the sauce over the ribs on each plate.

CHEFS NOTE
Pure canola oil is from rape seed and should therefore be gluten free. Although you can substitute in this recipe for any other oil you prefer.

ITALIAN STYLE ROAST

455 calories per serving

Ingredients

- 675g/1½lb braising steak
- 15 cloves garlic, finely sliced
- 4 sun-dried tomatoes, chopped
- 120ml/½ cup red wine
- 2 tbsp balsamic vinegar
- 1 tsp dried thyme
- ¼ tsp fresh black pepper
- 1 tsp arrowroot
- 2 tsp water
- 10 green olives, sliced

Method

1 Trim the beef to remove all visible fat and cube the meat.

2 Place the garlic and sun-dried tomatoes in the slow cooker. Lay the beef on top. Pour the wine over the meat, and sprinkle with the vinegar, thyme and black pepper.

3 Cook on Low for 6-7 hours, or until the meat is very tender. Remove the meat to a platter, and turn up the slow cooker to High.

4 In a small bowl, mix the arrowroot with 2 teaspoons of water to make a smooth paste. Add this to the liquid in the slow cooker, and stir.

5 Cover, and cook for 10 minutes or until the sauce has thickened. Pour the sauce over the meat, and stir in the sliced olives.

6 Serve over rice or noodles.

CHEFS NOTE
This tastes even better cooked the day before and refrigerated overnight.

THAI CHICKEN SOUP

285
calories per serving

Ingredients

- 2 tbsp red curry paste
- 750ml/3 cups unsweetened coconut milk
- 500ml/2 cups gluten free hot chicken stock
- 2 tbsp fish sauce
- 2 tbsp brown sugar
- 1 tbsp peanut butter
- 550g/1¼lb chicken breasts, cubed

- 1 red pepper, seeded and sliced
- 1 medium onion, peeled thinly sliced
- 1 tbsp root ginger, grated
- 150g/5oz frozen peas, thawed
- 1 tbsp lime juice
- 1 tbsp chopped coriander

Method

1 Combine together the curry paste, coconut milk, chicken stock, fish sauce, brown sugar and peanut butter in the slow cooker. Add the chicken breast, pepper, onion and ginger. Cover and cook on High for 4 hours.

2 Add in the peas and cook for a further 30 minutes or until everything is cooked through and piping hot. Stir in the lime juice and serve garnished with coriander.

CHEFS NOTE
Peanut butter is naturally gluten free. However there is potential for cross contamination during manufacture, so you may prefer to buy a brand labelled as gluten free.

CHICKEN WITH SALSA

374 calories per serving

Ingredients

- 750ml/3 cups salsa verde
- 500ml/2 cups gluten free hot vegetable stock
- 1.8kg/4lb whole chicken
- 1 onion, peeled & chopped
- 1 red pepper, seeded & chopped
- 1 bay leaf
- 1 tsp ground coriander
- 1 tbsp chopped fresh coriander
- Salt and pepper to taste

Method

1 Cut the chicken into 6 parts: 2 legs, 2 breasts and 2 wings. Discard the skin and any extra fat.

2 Add the salsa verde and the stock to the slow cooker. Add the chicken parts, the onion, pepper, bay leaf, and both the ground and fresh coriander. Stir well. Cook on High for 3-4 hours or on Low for 6-8 hours.

3 When the chicken is well cooked, remove it from the slow cooker. Take the meat off the bones and shred it with two forks. Discard the bones and put the shredded chicken back in the slow cooker.

4 Ladle into bowls and serve.

CHEFS NOTE
You can use shop-bought salsa verde or create your own by combining fresh tomatoes garlic, onion, coriander, jalapeños, limes juice, ground cumin, honey and salt.

SPLIT PEA AND HAM SOUP

355 calories per serving

Ingredients

- 450g/1lb dried green split peas
- 1 tbsp olive oil
- 1 onion, chopped
- 2 stalks celery, chopped
- 2 carrots, chopped
- 2 cloves garlic, crushed

- 2 ham hocks
- 1½lt/6 cups of water
- 2 tsp fresh thyme, chopped
- 2 tsp fresh sage, chopped
- Salt and pepper

Method

1 Heat the olive oil in a large pan over a medium heat. Sauté the onion, celery and carrots for a few minutes until softened. Add the garlic and cook for another minute. Remove from the heat and put into the slow cooker.

2 Add the peas, water and ham hocks to the slow cooker along with the herbs, salt and pepper.

3 Combine well, cover and cook on High for 4-5 hours, or on Low for 8-10 hours, until the ham falls off the bone.

4 Remove the bones, using forks to shred off any reaming meat. Adjust the seasoning and spoon into bowls.

CHEFS NOTE
Ham hocks are readily available from butcher's counters.

POTATOES WITH CHEESE AND BACON

320 calories per serving

Ingredients

- 4 slices of back bacon
- 1.35kg/3lb potatoes, scrubbed and sliced (no need to peel)
- 150g/5oz mature Cheddar cheese, grated
- ½ tbsp mixed herbs
- 1 tbsp chives, chopped

Method

1 Grill the bacon until crispy, allow it to cool then finely chop.

2 Line the slow cooker with aluminium foil, leaving enough spare to wrap over the top of the potatoes. Coat the foil with cooking spray.

3 Place a layer of potatoes evenly on the bottom of the slow cooker. Sprinkle on some of the cheese, herbs and bacon, repeating twice more.

4 Cover the potatoes with the aluminium foil flaps. Put the lid on and cook on Low for 7-8 hours or on High for 3-4 hours.

5 Serve immediately, garnished with the chives and a little extra grated cheese.

CHEFS NOTE

This is also good using a combination of cheddar and blue cheese.

CHICKEN AND RICE

292 calories per serving

Ingredients

- 1 tbsp extra-virgin olive oil
- 1 onion, finely chopped
- 1 red pepper, seeded & chopped
- 225g/8oz rice
- 250g/9oz chicken breast, cubed
- 250ml/1 cup gluten free hot chicken stock
- 400g/14oz tin chopped tomatoes
- ½ tsp freshly ground black pepper
- ½ tsp cayenne pepper
- ½ tsp chilli flakes
- Salt

Method

Heat the oil in a large pan, and sauté the onions and pepper for a few minutes until softened. Add the rice and continue to cook for another couple of minutes.

Add all the ingredients to the slow cooker. Cover and cook on Low for 4 hours or until the chicken and rice are both cooked through and tender.

CHEFS NOTE

Adjust the quantities of cayenne pepper and chilli flakes to suit your own heat preference!

HAWAIIAN CHICKEN

254 calories per serving

Ingredients

- 675g/1½lb chicken breasts, cubed
- 2 red peppers, seeded & sliced
- 550g/1¼lb tin pineapple chunks in natural juice
- 2 tbsp gluten free soy sauce
- 2 cloves garlic, crushed
- 2 tsp freshly grated ginger
- 1 tbsp honey
- 2 tsp cornstarch

Method

1 Pour the juice from the pineapple chunks into a small mixing bowl.

2 Add the soy sauce, garlic, ginger and honey, and whisk together. Add the cornstarch and stir well.

3 Place the chicken in the slow cooker. Pour the juice mixture and the pineapple chunks over the chicken along with the peppers. Cover and cook on Low for 4-5 hours.

CHEFS NOTE
Feel free to add some green beans or vegetables to this sweet dish and serve with rice if you wish.

EASY CHILLI CON CARNE

390
calories per
serving

Ingredients

- 1 tsp olive oil
- 500g/1lb 2oz lean beef mince
- 1 onion, chopped
- 2 tbsp tomato puree/paste
- 400g/14oz tin tomatoes
- 1 green chilli, seeded & chopped
- 2 tsp chilli powder
- Salt and pepper
- ½ tsp ground cumin
- 400g/14oz tin kidney beans, drained
- ½ tbsp unsweetened cocoa powder
- 500ml/2 cups hot beef stock

Method

1 Heat the oil in a frying pan and brown the mince & chopped onion in a large pan for a few minutes.

2 Drain off any fat and add all the ingredients into the slow cooker. Cover and cook on Low for 6-8 hours or High for 3-4 hours.

CHEFS NOTE
Add some tinned sweetcorn to the slow cooker if you wish. Perfect served with brown rice.

THE *Skinny* *gluten free* SLOW COOKER

RECIPE BOOK

Fish & Seafood

SMOKED HADDOCK CHOWDER

315 calories per serving

Ingredients

- Knob of butter
- 3 rashers of streaky bacon, chopped
- 1½ onions, finely sliced
- 750ml/3 cups milk
- 5 medium potatoes, peeled & finely chopped
- 400g/14oz boneless smoked haddock fillets
- 200g/7oz sweetcorn
- 1 tbsp chopped flat leaf parsley

Method

1 Heat the butter in a frying pan and sauté the bacon, potatoes and onions for a few minutes until the onions are soft.

2 Add to the slow cooker along with milk and cook on High for about an hour.

3 Stir in the sweetcorn and lay the fish on top. Cover and cook for another 25 minutes, or until the fish is cooked through and flakes easily. Sprinkle chopped parsley over the top and serve.

CHEFS NOTE
Add stock to alter the consistency.

PEA AND PRAWN CURRY

237
calories per serving

Ingredients

- 1 tbsp vegetable oil
- 2 onions, peeled & cut into wedges
- 6 ripe tomatoes, quartered
- 1 tsp fresh root ginger, grated
- 6 cloves garlic, crushed

- 3 tbsp curry paste
- 400g/14oz shelled raw king prawns
- 250g/9oz frozen peas
- 1 tbsp chopped fresh coriander

Method

1 Heat the oil in frying pan and sauté the onions over a medium heat until soft.

2 Combine everything in the slow cooker, except the prawns, peas & fresh coriander. Cover and cook on High for 3 hours.

3 After this time add the prawns and peas. Cover and cook for a further 45-60 minutes, or until the prawns are pink and cooked through.

4 Scatter the chopped coriander over the top and serve.

CHEFS NOTE
Serve with spiced Basmati rice.

FISH AND PAPRIKA

276 calories per serving

Ingredients

- 1 tbsp chopped flat-leaf parsley
- 1 tbsp olive oil
- Pinch of salt and pepper
- 2 onions, thinly sliced
- 1 garlic clove, crushed
- 2 stalks celery, finely chopped

- 2 tsp smoked paprika
- 200g/7oz roasted red peppers from a jar, drained & sliced
- 400g/14oz tin chopped tomato
- 600g/1lb 5oz boneless white fish fillet, cut into large chunks

Method

1 Heat the oil in a pan and gently sauté the onions, garlic and celery for a few minutes until softened. Add this to the slow cooker along with the paprika, peppers and tomatoes. Cover and cook on Low for 3-4 hours.

2 Lay the fish on top. Re-cover and cook on High for around 45 minutes. Stir the fish into the sauce then serve with chopped parsley sprinkled over the top.

CHEFS NOTE
Serve with your choice of green vegetables, potatoes and/or gluten free bread.

CHEAT'S FISH STEW

280 calories per serving

Ingredients

- 900g/2lb firm white fish fillets
- 400g/14oz tin tomato soup
- 400g/14oz tin chopped tomatoes
- 1 onion, peeled and chopped
- 2 red peppers, seeded & sliced
- 500ml/2 cups gluten free hot fish stock
- Salt and pepper
- 1 tbsp ground mixed herbs
- 1 bay leaf

Method

1 Add all the ingredients to your slow cooker. Combine well, cover and cook on Low for 4-6 hours. Remove the bay leaf, adjust the seasoning, and serve.

CHEFS NOTE

Any type of firm of white fish, works with this simple recipe.

SIMPLE HAKE

140 calories per serving

Ingredients

- 650g/1lb 7oz hake fillet, skinned, cut into chunks
- 3 cloves garlic, crushed
- 120ml/½ cup gluten free hot chicken stock
- 25ml/1fl oz lemon juice
- Salt and pepper to taste
- 1 tbsp chopped chives

Method

1 Place the fish in the slow cooker. In a bowl combine the garlic, chicken stock, lemon juice, salt and pepper, then pour the mixture over fish. Cover and cook on High for 1-2 hours or until the fish is cooked through and easily flakes with a fork.

2 Remove the fillets, season with plenty of freshly ground black pepper and sprinkled chives.

CHEFS NOTE
Great served with mashed potatoes and steamed greens.

COD AND PRAWN CHOWDER

303
calories per serving

Ingredients

- 1 tsp oil
- 4 slices of back bacon, chopped
- 1 onion, chopped
- 2 cloves garlic, crushed
- 1lt/4 cups gluten free hot chicken stock
- 175g/6oz sweetcorn
- 2 large potatoes, peeled and cubed

- 3 stalks celery, chopped
- 2 large carrots, peeled and chopped
- Salt & pepper to taste
- ½ tsp Cayenne pepper
- 350g/12oz peeled king prawns,
- 125g/4oz cod fillet, skinned, chopped
- 120ml/½ cup evaporated milk

Method

1 Heat the oil and fry the bacon, onions and garlic for a few minutes. Add the carrots & celery and sauté for another couple of minutes.

2 Transfer both the vegetables and bacon to the slow cooker. Add the stock, corn, potatoes and cayenne pepper. Season with black pepper. Cover and cook on High for 2 hours.

3 Add the shrimp and the cod, re-cover and cook for a further 15 minutes. Pour in the evaporated milk and heat through for another 30 minutes or until the seafood is cooked through.

CHEFS NOTE

Use any type of firm white fish you prefer for this thick soup.

SEAFOOD STEW

210 calories per serving

Ingredients

- 1 tbsp olive oil
- 2 cloves garlic, crushed
- 150g/5oz carrots, finely chopped
- 600g/1lb5oz fresh tomatoes, sliced
- 1 green pepper, seeded & chopped
- ½ tsp fennel seeds
- 500ml/2 cups gluten free hot fish or chicken stock

- 450g/1lb cod fillets, cubed
- 225g/8oz king prawns, peeled
- 1 tsp dried basil
- 1 tsp brown sugar
- ½ tsp salt
- Few drops Tabasco sauce
- 2 tbsp chopped fresh flat leaf parsley

Method

1 Mix the oil and garlic in the slow cooker. Add the carrots, tomatoes, peppers, fennel seeds, & stock.

2 Combine well, cover and cook on Low for 4 hours, or until the vegetables are tender.

3 About 20 minutes before the end of cooking time, gently stir in the cod, prawns, sugar, basil, salt, and Tabasco. Cover again, and cook on High for 20-30 minutes or until the seafood is cooked through.

4 Sprinkle with parsley and serve.

CHEFS NOTE
Although Tabasco sauce contains vinegar there is no detectable gluten in the finished product.

CIOPPINO

387
calories per
serving

Ingredients

- 1 tbsp olive oil
- 2 onions, sliced
- ½ fennel bulb, chopped
- 10 garlic cloves, finely sliced
- 250ml/1 cup dry white wine
- 2 tsp tomato puree
- 120ml/½ cup gluten free hot fish stock
- 2 tbsp fresh oregano, chopped
- 2 tbsp fresh thyme, chopped
- ¾ tsp chilli flakes
- ½ tsp sea salt
- 2 x 400g/14oz tin chopped tomatoes
- 350g/12oz cod fillets, cubed
- 350g/12oz king prawns, peeled
- 1 tbsp lemon juice
- 1 tbsp chopped fresh basil

Method

1 Heat the oil in a large pan. Sauté the onion, fennel, and garlic for around 3 minutes, until soft. Stir in the wine and tomato puree and bring to the boil. Cook for another couple of minutes, stirring occasionally.

2 Pour the onion mixture into the slow cooker. Add the water, oregano, thyme, chilli flakes, salt and tinned tomatoes. Cover and cook on Low for 7 hours.

3 Stir in the cod, scallops, shrimp, and lemon juice. Cover and cook on Low for around 30 minutes, or until the seafood is properly cooked through.

4 Serve garnished with fresh basil.

CHEFS NOTE

This dish can be made with a wide variety of fish and shellfish, so feel free to experiment!

SALMON WITH SPINACH

267
calories per serving

Ingredients

- 350g/12oz fresh spinach
- 675g/1½lb salmon
- Salt and pepper to taste
- 2 tsp ground dill
- 2 lemons, sliced
- 60ml/¼ cup gluten free hot fish stock

Method

1 Add the spinach to the slow cooker. Place the salmon on top, sprinkled on each side with the salt, pepper and dill.

2 Place the sliced lemons over the top of the fish and add the stock.

3 Cook on Low for 2 hours, or until the fish is cooked through and flakes easily with a fork.

CHEFS NOTE
Serve with a green salad or boiled new potatoes.

HONEY TILAPIA

300
calories per serving

Ingredients

- 600g/1lb 5oz tilapia filets
- 2 tbsp balsamic vinegar
- 1 tbsp honey
- 300g/11oz tinned mandarin oranges, drained
- Salt and pepper to taste

Method

1 Line the inside of the slow cooker with tin foil leaving enough overhang to cover the fish.

2 Place the tilapia fillets in the middle, drizzle the balsamic vinegar and honey over and place the mandarin oranges on top.

3 Fold the foil over and turn the edges to make a parcel. Cook on High for 2 hours, or until the fish is cooked through flakes easily with a fork. Season to taste with some salt and pepper.

CHEFS NOTE

Great served with plenty of steamed tenderstem broccoli.

SUPER EASY PESTO SOLE

323 calories per serving

Ingredients

- 675g/1½lb sole fillets
- 150g/5oz pesto
- 1 tbsp Parmesan cheese, grated

Method

1 Line the inside of the slow cooker with tin foil leaving enough overhang to cover the fish.

2 Place the sole fillets in the middle spread the pesto over the top of each and sprinkle on a little grated Parmesan. Fold the foil over and turn the edges to make a parcel.

3 Cover and cook on Low for 3-4 hours. Check the fish after 3 hours. When it is fully white and flakes easily with a fork, it is ready.

CHEFS NOTE

Buy labelled gluten free Pesto to ensure you are safe from cross contamination.

THE *Skinny* gluten free SLOW COOKER

RECIPE BOOK

Vegetable/Vegetarian

LENTIL AND CARROT SOUP

235 calories per serving

Ingredients

- 2 tbsp olive oil
- 600g/1lb 5oz carrots, washed & grated (no need to peel)
- 140g/4½oz split red lentils, rinsed
- 1lt/4 cups gluten free hot vegetable stock
- 2 tsp cumin seeds
- 1 tsp chilli flakes
- 120ml/½ cup milk
- Natural yogurt, to serve

Method

1 Place the oil, carrots, lentils and stock into the slow cooker. Add half the cumin seeds and half the chilli flakes. Cover and cook on High for 2-3 hours or until the lentils are tender.

2 Dry-fry the remaining cumin seeds and chilli flakes until just fragrant.

3 When the soup is cooked, stir in the milk and blend until you have your preferred consistency. Serve sprinkled with the toasted spices.

CHEFS NOTE
Add more stock or milk if you want to alter the consistency.

PESTO MUSHROOMS WITH RICOTTA

320
calories per serving

Ingredients

- 2 tbsp extra-virgin olive oil
- 28 medium chestnut mushrooms
- 250g/9oz tub low fat ricotta cheese
- 2 tbsp green pesto, + 1 tbsp to serve
- 2 cloves garlic, peeled and finely chopped
- 1 tbsp Parmesan cheese, grated
- 2 tbsp chopped fresh flat leaf parsley, to serve

Method

1 Generously brush the inside of the slow cooker with 1 tbsp of the oil. Trim the mushroom stalks, then place the mushrooms, rounded cap side down, in the slow cooker.

2 In a bowl, mix together the ricotta, pesto and garlic, and spoon the mixture over the mushrooms. Sprinkle the Parmesan over the top and then drizzle on the rest of the oil.

3 Cook on Low for 6-8 hours. Drain off any excess juice.

4 To serve, blob a little more pesto on top of each mushroom and scatter with the parsley.

CHEFS NOTE
Pesto is naturally gluten free, being traditionally made from fresh basil, Parmesan cheese, pine nuts, olive oil and garlic.

MEDITERRANEAN VEGETABLE BAKE

310 calories per serving

····· *Ingredients* ·····

- 4 cloves garlic, crushed
- 400g/14oz tin chopped tomatoes
- 1 tsp fresh oregano leaves, chopped
- Large pinch chilli flakes
- Salt and pepper
- 1 aubergine, sliced

- 2 courgettes, sliced
- 2 roasted red peppers, chopped
- 3 large beef tomatoes, sliced
- 1 tbsp fresh basil, chopped
- 2 gluten free white ciabatta rolls, quartered
- 225g/8oz low fat mozzarella cheese, sliced

····· *Method* ·····

1 In a bowl mix together the tinned tomatoes, crushed garlic, oregano leaves & chilli.

2 Add half of this to the slow cooker then layer over half the aubergines, courgettes, red peppers, tomatoes & basil. Lay half the bread on top of this along half the mozzarella slices.

3 Now add the rest of the tinned tomatoes mixture to the slow cooker and layer over the rest of the veg, bread and mozzarella,

4 Push everything down well, cover and cook on High for 5-6 hours.

5 Serve with a large green salad.

CHEFS NOTE
Shop-bought roasted peppers are a handy store cupboard ingredient.

VEGETABLE TAGINE

274 calories per serving

Ingredients

- 4 medium carrots, roughly chopped
- 4 small parsnips, roughly chopped
- 3 red onions, peeled and cut into wedges
- 2 red peppers, seeded and chopped
- 2 tbsp olive oil
- 1 tsp each ground cumin

- 1 tsp ground paprika
- 1 tsp ground cinnamon
- 1 tsp mild chilli powder
- 400g/14oz tin chopped tomatoes
- 50g/2oz dried apricot
- 2 tsp honey

Method

1 Combine all the ingredients well in the slow cooker.

2 Cover and cook on Low for 6-8 hours or until the vegetables are tender.

3 This is great as it is or you could also serve with quinoa or brown rice.

CHEFS NOTE

This simple recipe provides all your five-a-day in one tasty meal!

VEGETARIAN SHEPHERD'S PIE

498 calories per serving

Ingredients

For the lentil sauce:
- 25g/1oz butter
- 1 onion, peeled and chopped
- 2 medium carrots, peeled and chopped
- 2 stalks celery, chopped
- 2 cloves garlic, crushed
- 100g/3½oz chestnut mushroom, sliced
- 1 bay leaf
- ½ tbsp dried thyme
- 250g/9oz dried green lentils, rinsed

- 60ml/¼ cup red wine
- 750ml/3 cups gluten free hot vegetable stock
- 1½ tbsp tomato purée
- Salt and pepper

For the topping:
- 1kg/2¼lb floury potatoes
- 40g/1½oz butter
- 60ml/¼ cup milk
- Salt and pepper
- 25g/1oz Cheddar cheese, grated

Method

1 Heat the butter in a frying pan, and sauté the onions, carrots, celery and garlic for about 10 minutes until soft. Add these to your slow cooker along with the mushrooms, herbs, tomato puree & lentils. Pour in the stock and wine, cover and cook on High for 5-6 hours.

2 After a few hours of cooking, boil the potatoes in a pan of salted water for about 15 minutes until they're cooked. Drain and mash with butter and milk. Season with salt and pepper.

3 Top with the mashed potato, sprinkle on the cheese, and cook for another 30 minutes until piping hot.

CHEFS NOTE

You can also make individual pies by dividing the mixture between dishes before you add the mashed potato. These can also be frozen for a later date – for best results, defrost before re-heating.

GARLIC MUSHROOM SPAGHETTI

345 calories per serving

Ingredients

- 2 tbsp olive oil
- 250g/9oz chestnut mushrooms, thickly sliced
- 1 clove garlic, peeled and thinly sliced
- 1 tbsp chopped flat leaf parsley
- 1 stalk celery, finely chopped
- 1 medium onion, finely chopped
- 400g/14oz tin chopped tomatoes
- ½ red chilli, seeded & finely chopped
- 300g/11oz gluten free spaghetti

Method

1 Add all the ingredients except the parsley and pasta to your slow cooker. Cover and cook on Low for 6-7 hours.

2 15 minutes before you're ready to eat, cook the spaghetti in salted boiling water.

3 Drain and toss with the cooked mushrooms. Scatter with parsley, and serve.

CHEFS NOTE
Gluten free pasta is made with corn and rice instead of wheat.

VEGETABLE KORMA

320 calories per serving

Ingredients

- 1 tbsp vegetable oil
- 1 onion, finely chopped
- 3 cardamom pods, bashed
- 2 tsp ground cumin
- 2 tsp ground coriander
- ½ tsp ground turmeric
- 1 green chilli, seeded & finely chopped
- 1 clove garlic, crushed
- 1 tsp grated root ginger
- 800g/1¾lb mixed vegetables (e.gs carrots, cauliflower, potato, courgette), chopped
- 500ml/2 cups gluten free hot vegetable stock
- 200g/7oz peas
- 250ml/1 cup fat free Greek yoghurt
- 2 tbsp ground almonds
- 1 tbsp chopped coriander

Method

1 Heat the oil in a frying pan and gently sauté the onions with the dry spices for a few minutes. Add the chilli, garlic and ginger and cook for a further minute or two and then scrape into the slow cooker.

2 Add all the vegetables and the stock. Cover and cook on Low for 4-5 hours or until the potatoes are tender.

3 Stir in the peas and cook for a further 10 minutes. Stir through the yoghurt and serve sprinkled with fresh coriander.

CHEFS NOTE
Any vegetables will work with this recipe, so use your favourites or whatever you have to hand!

CHICKPEA AND BUTTERNUT SQUASH CURRY

336 calories per serving

Ingredients

- 550g/1¼lb butternut squash, peeled, seeded & cubed
- 150g/5oz dried chickpeas, rinsed
- 1 onion, chopped
- 1 clove garlic, crushed
- 250ml/1 cup light coconut milk
- 100g/3½oz fresh spinach, roughly chopped
- 165g/5½oz peas
- 1 large tomato, diced
- 400ml/14fl oz gluten free hot vegetable stock
- 1½ tbsp curry powder
- 1 tsp salt
- 25g/1oz fresh coriander, roughly chopped

Method

1 Add all the ingredients except the peas and spinach to the slow cooker.

2 Cook on High for 5-6 hours or until the chickpeas are tender.

3 About 20-30 minutes before serving add in the peas and spinach, and stir. Re-cover and leave to finish cooking.

CHEFS NOTE

If your sauce is a little too thin at the end, make a paste of cornstarch and hot water and stir a little into the slow cooker until it thickens.

PUMPKIN RISOTTO

Ingredients

- 3 tbsp olive oil
- 2 cloves garlic, crushed
- 1 leek, thinly sliced
- 1 onion, chopped
- 1 red pepper, seeded & chopped
- 180ml/¾ cup dry white wine
- 500g/1lb2oz Arborio rice

- 1 tsp sea salt
- 1lt/4 cups gluten free hot vegetable stock
- 1 tbsp fresh thyme, split in half.
- 250ml/1 cup pumpkin puree
- 1 tbsp olive oil
- 1 small pumpkin, seeded, peeled & cubed
- Salt and pepper

Method

1 Heat the olive oil in a pan over medium-high heat and sauté the leeks, onions and red pepper for about a few minutes. Add the garlic and cook for another minute.

2 Place the contents of the pan in the slow cooker along with the wine, rice, stock, salt and half of the fresh thyme.

3 Cover and cook on High for about 2-3 hours or until all the liquid is absorbed.

4 While the risotto is cooking, roast the pumpkin. Preheat the oven to 425°F/220C. Toss the pumpkin cubes with olive oil and a little salt, and roast for 30-40 minutes or until lightly browned and tender. Remove from the oven and set aside.

5 Just before serving, stir the pumpkin puree, roasted pumpkin and the remaining thyme into the slow cooker. Cover and leave for another 5 minutes before serving.

CHEFS NOTE

Pumpkin puree is high in fibre and gluten free.

LENTIL, SPINACH AND SWEET POTATO SOUP

193 calories per serving

Ingredients

- 1 onion, chopped
- 1 stalk celery, chopped
- 1 carrot, thinly sliced
- 1 leek, sliced
- 2 cloves garlic, crushed
- 1 large sweet potato, peeled and cubed
- 100g/3½oz green lentils, soaked and rinsed

- 1lt/4 cups gluten free hot vegetable stock
- ½ tbsp gluten free soy sauce
- 1 bay leaf
- ½ tbsp fresh rosemary, roughly chopped
- 200g/7oz fresh baby spinach.
- Sea salt and freshly ground black pepper, to taste

Method

1 After soaking the lentils, discard the soaking water and rinse the beans in a strainer. Add rinsed beans and all of the other ingredients except the spinach to the slow cooker.

2 Combine well, cover and cook on Low for 6-8 hours or until the lentils are tender.

3 A few minutes before serving stir in the fresh spinach. Season with salt and pepper to taste and serve.

CHEFS NOTE
If you prefer a smooth soup, blend before serving.

CURRIED COCONUT AND VEGETABLE SOUP

354 calories per serving

Ingredients

- 1 small onion, diced
- 1 leek, thinly sliced
- 2 cloves garlic, crushed
- 1 tsp fresh root ginger, grated
- 225g/8oz butternut squash, peeled, seeded & diced
- 225g/8oz parsnips, chopped
- 750ml/3 cups gluten free hot vegetable stock
- 1½ tbsp red curry paste

- ½ tbsp gluten free tamari sauce
- 75g/3oz peas
- 100g/3½oz kale, stems removed & roughly chopped
- 180ml/¾ cup light coconut milk
- Juice from ½ lime
- Sea salt, to taste
- 2 spring onions, chopped
- 1 tbsp fresh chopped coriander

Method

1 Add the onions, leeks, garlic, ginger, squash, parsnips, stock & paste to the slow cooker. Combine well, cover and cook on High for 4 to 6 hours, or on Low for 8 hours.

2 About 30 minutes before the end of the cooking time add the kale, peas, coconut milk and lime juice. Stir and cook for a further 30 minutes or until everything is tender and piping hot.

3 Serve garnished with coriander and spring onions.

CHEFS NOTE

Like soy sauce, tamari is made from soya beans and is traditionally gluten free. However, some brands may in fact contain wheat, so you should always check the label.

CREAMY POTATO SOUP

245 calories per serving

Ingredients

- 1 tbsp olive oil
- 1 onion, finely chopped
- 1 clove garlic, crushed
- 450g/1lb potatoes, peeled & diced
- 500ml/2 cups skimmed milk, (+ 2 tbsp reserved for later)
- 500ml/2 cups gluten free hot vegetable stock
- 1 tbsp fresh rosemary, chopped
- Salt and pepper to taste
- ¼ tsp paprika
- 2 tbsp cornstarch

Method

1 Heat the oil in a small pan and gently sauté the onion & garlic for a few minutes.

2 Add the to the slow cooker along with the milk, stock, rosemary, salt, pepper & paprika.

3 Combine well, cover and cook on Low for 6 to 8 hours or until everything is tender and cooked though.

4 About 15 minutes before the end of cooking time, combine the cornstarch with the reserved 2 tbsp milk in a small bowl, and stir until smooth. Add the mixture to the slow cooker, stirring. Cover again and cook for another 15 minutes or until the sauce has thickened.

CHEFS NOTE
If you prefer a smooth consistency, blend before serving.

SIMPLE VEGETABLE STEW

180 calories per serving

Ingredients

- 1 onion, peeled and chopped
- 2 stalks celery, chopped
- 1 large sweet potato, cubed
- 3 medium carrots, chopped
- 225g/8oz butternut squash, peeled, seeded & cubed
- 150g/5oz green beans

- Salt and pepper
- Pinch chilli flakes
- 1 tbsp fresh thyme
- 370ml/ 1½ cups gluten free hot vegetable stock
- 500ml/2 cups semi-skimmed milk

Method

1 Add all the ingredients, except the milk to the slow cooker.

2 Cover and cook on Low for 8-9 hours, or until the carrots are tender.

3 In the last 30 minutes of cooking time, stir in the milk, re-cover and continue cooking.

4 Serve with crusty gluten free bread.

CHEFS NOTE

If you find the sauce too thin, thicken with a little cornstarch and water when you add the milk.

LENTIL AND VEGETABLE STEW

294 calories per serving

Ingredients

- 175g/6oz sweetcorn
- 1 large potato, diced
- 4 carrots, diced
- 1 onion, chopped
- 2 stalks celery, sliced
- 150g/5oz fresh green beans
- ½ tsp paprika
- Salt and pepper
- 370ml/1½ cups tomato passata/sieved tomatoes
- 750ml/3 cups gluten free hot vegetable stock
- 200g/7oz lentils, rinsed

Method

1 Add all of the ingredients to the slow cooker. Stir, cover and cook on Low for 8-10 hours or until everything is tender and cooked through.

2 When the time is up, if you find the stew too thin, cook for another half hour on High with the lid off.

CHEFS NOTE

Feel free to add or substitute vegetables according to what you have or what you like – it works with pretty much any veg!

SPICED SWEET POTATO MASH

222 calories per serving

Ingredients

- 900g/2lb sweet potatoes, peeled & sliced
- 250ml/1 cup fresh apple juice
- 1 tsp ground cinnamon
- ½ tsp ground nutmeg
- ½ tsp allspice
- ¼ tsp ground cloves
- Pinch of cinnamon and nutmeg to garnish
- 25g/1oz pecan nuts, shelled, to garnish

Method

1 Tip the sweet potatoes into the slow cooker. Add half of the apple juice and the dry spices.

2 Cook on Low for 4-5 hours or until the potatoes are tender.

3 Combine the sweet potatoes, with the remaining apple juice. Season and serve with a sprinkling of pecans.

CHEFS NOTE
The nuts add a welcome texture to this dish try chopped pistachios or cashews too.

CHEESY PASTA

301 calories per serving

Ingredients

- 250ml/1 cup skimmed milk
- 2 egg whites
- 2 tsp cornstarch
- 125g/4oz low fat mature Cheddar cheese
- 300g/11oz gluten free pasta, preferably penne

Method

1 Whisk together the milk, egg whites & cornstarch and add these to the slow cooker along with the cheese and pasta.

2 Cook on Low for 1½-2 hours or until the pasta of tender.

3 Stir occasionally and serve.

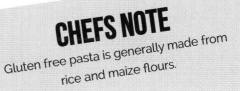

CHEFS NOTE
Gluten free pasta is generally made from rice and maize flours.

MUSHROOM PILAF

270
calories per
serving

Ingredients

- 225g/8oz rice
- ½ tbsp olive oil
- 500ml/2 cups gluten free hot vegetable stock
- 4 shallots, finely chopped
- 250g/9oz mushrooms, sliced

- 1 clove garlic, crushed
- ½ tbsp fresh rosemary, chopped
- ½ tbsp fresh sage, chopped
- 1 tsp fresh thyme, chopped

Method

1 Gently combine the rice and olive oil together in the slow cooker until the rice is coated with the oil.

2 Add the stock, shallots, mushrooms, garlic, and herbs.

3 Stir well, cover and cook on Low for 5 hours or until the rice is tender and the stock has been absorbed.

CHEFS NOTE
You may need to increase/decrease the amount of stock you use to get the consistency right.

BUTTERNUT SQUASH SOUP

217
calories per
serving

Ingredients

- 675g/1½lb butternut squash, peeled, seeded & diced
- 1 large potato, cubed
- 1 red pepper, seeded & chopped
- 100g/3½oz sweetcorn
- 200g/7oz tinned black beans, rinsed and drained
- 200g/7oz tinned haricot beans, rinsed and drained
- 200g/7oz tinned chopped tomatoes
- 1 onion, finely chopped
- 750ml/3 cups gluten free hot vegetable stock
- 1 tbsp chopped coriander
- ¼ tsp cayenne pepper
- ¼ tsp ginger
- ¼ tsp cumin
- ¼ tsp ground black pepper
- 1 jalapeño chilli, diced, seeded if desired

Method

1 Combine all the ingredients in the slow cooker except the chopped coriander and diced chilli.

2 Cover and cook on Low for 6-8 hours or until everything is tender and cooked through.

3 Serve sprinkled with a little fresh coriander and chilli.

CHEFS NOTE

If you prefer a smoother soup, blend half the soup after cooking and stir through half a cup of milk or a little crème fraiche.

SUPERFOOD SOUP

217 calories per serving

Ingredients

- 150g/5oz carrots, sliced
- 1 small sweet potato, cubed
- 75g/3oz green beans
- 1 tbsp chopped fresh coriander
- 1 onion, diced
- 1 clove garlic, crushed
- 400g/14oz tin black beans, drained & rinsed
- ¼ tsp chilli flakes
- ¼ tsp black pepper
- ½ tsp chilli powder
- ½ tsp ground cumin
- Sea salt to taste
- 250ml/1 cup vegetable juice
- 500ml/2 cups gluten free hot vegetable stock

Method

1 Combine all the ingredients in the slow cooker.

2 Cover and cook on Low for 6-8 hours or until everything is tender and piping hot.

3 Remove two ladles of soup from the slow cooker and put to one side.

4 Blend the remaining soup and combine with the reserved soup.

CHEFS NOTE
Serve with crusty gluten free bread.

SERVES 4

EDAMAME AND SQUASH KORMA

320 calories per serving

Ingredients

- 1 tbsp vegetable oil
- 1 onion, peeled & chopped
- 4 cardamom pods, squashed
- 2 tsp ground cumin
- 2 tsp ground coriander
- 1 tsp ground turmeric
- 1 green chilli, seeded and finely chopped
- 1 clove garlic, peeled and crushed
- 1 tbsp grated root ginger

- 450g/1lb butternut squash, peeled, seeded & cubed
- 1 small cauliflower, broken into large florets
- 1 red pepper, deseeded & roughly chopped
- 500ml/2 cups hot vegetable stock
- 200g/7oz edamame beans
- 150g/5oz fat free Greek plain yogurt
- 2 tbsp ground almonds
- 2 tbsp flaked almonds, toasted

Method

1 Heat the oil in a large pan, and gently sauté the onion and spices over a low heat for a few minutes until softened. Add the chilli, garlic and ginger, cook for another minute and then empty the pan into the slow cooker.

2 Add the squash, cauliflower and pepper, and pour in the stock. Cook on Low for 4 hours.

3 Stir in the beans and edemame and ground almonds. Season with salt and pepper, and leave for 10 minutes to heat through.

4 Stir through the yoghurt, scatter with flaked almonds & coriander leaves.

CHEFS NOTE
Serve with long grain or cauliflower 'rice' and gluten free naan bread.

MUSHROOM AND BLACK BEAN CHILLI

310 calories per serving

Ingredients

- 225g/8oz black beans, rinsed
- ½ tbsp extra-virgin olive oil
- 1 tsp mustard seeds
- 1 tbsp chilli powder
- 1 tsp cumin seeds
- ¼ tsp cardamom seeds
- 1 onion, chopped
- 225g/8oz mushrooms, sliced
- 125g/4oz tomatoes, roughly chopped
- 2 tbsp water

- 750ml/3 cups gluten free hot vegetable stock
- 2 tbsp tomato puree
- 1 jalapeño chilli, seeded & chopped
- 75g/3oz reduced fat mature Cheddar cheese, grated
- 2 tbsp reduced-fat sour cream
- 1 tbsp chopped fresh coriander
- 1 lime, cut into wedges
- A few sprigs of coriander

Method

1 Soak the beans overnight and drain.

2 In a large pan, combine the oil, mustard seeds, chilli powder, cumin and cardamom. Cook over a high heat, stirring, until the spices sizzle, about 30 seconds. Add the onion, mushrooms, tomatoes and water. Cover and cook for another few minutes.

3 Add the stock, tomato puree and chilli.

4 Place the beans in the slow cooker along with the hot vegetables and stock from the pan. Combine well, cover and cook on high for 5-8 hours, or until the beans are tender and cooked through.

5 Serve garnished with cheese & chopped coriander, along with a dollop of sour cream and a wedge of lime.

CHEFS NOTE

If you don't have time to soak dried beans overnight just use tinned.

THE *Skinny* *gluten free* **SLOW COOKER**

RECIPE BOOK

Desserts

ROSEWATER APRICOTS

Ingredients

- 800g/1¾lb ripe apricots, halved & stoned
- 100g/3½oz caster sugar
- 180ml/¾ cup water

- A few drops rosewater
- 1 tbsp Greek yogurt, to serve
- 50g/2oz pistachios, roughly chopped

Method

1 Place the apricots in your slow cooker. Sprinkle on the sugar and add the water. Cover and cook on Low for 2 hours or until the apricots are soft and cooked through.

2 Place into a clean bowl, splash in the rosewater and leave to cool. Spoon into glasses and top with a teaspoon of yoghurt, sprinkled with the chopped pistachio nuts.

CHEFS NOTE

Once cooled, the poached apricots can be frozen for later.

APPLE CRUMBLE

447
calories per serving

Ingredients

- 1.1kg/2½lb eating apples
- 3 tbsp apricot jam
- Juice of 1 large orange
- For the crumble:
- 140g/4½oz gluten free oats
- 100g/3½oz gluten free flour
- 1 tsp ground cinnamon
- 100g/3½oz butter
- 100g/3½oz light muscovado sugar
- 1 tbsp golden syrup

Method

1 Peel, core and thinly slice the apples. Place them in the slow cooker and combine with the jam and orange juice. Cook on Low for 2-4 hours or until tender and cooked through.

2 When the apples are nearly done, mix the crumble ingredients in a baking tray and toast under a low grill for a couple of minutes, until golden.

3 According to your preference, either transfer the apples to a clean dish or leave them in the slow cooker pot. Scatter the crumble over the top.

4 Serve with your choice of cream or ice cream.

CHEFS NOTE

Gluten free flour can be made from many different sources, including rice, potato, tapioca, maize, buckwheat and corn, or from a blend of several ingredients. Any is suitable for this recipe.

APPLE AND PEAR COMPOTE

211 calories per serving

Ingredients

- 4 eating apples, peeled, cored & chopped
- 2 medium cooking apples, peeled, cored & chopped
- 4 firm pears, peeled, cored & sliced
- 100g/3½oz dried cherries
- 3 tbsp brown sugar
- 120ml/½ cup water

Method

1 Place the apples, pears, cherries and sugar into the slow cooker.

2 Add the water and combine well. Cover and cook on Low for 8-10 hours or until and the pears and apples are tender.

3 Divide into bowls and serve.

CHEFS NOTE
Try using cranberries instead of cherries if you prefer.

CHOCOLATE FUDGE

190
calories per serving

Ingredients

- 225g/8oz cups gluten free chocolate chips
- 60ml/¼ cup light coconut milk
- 25g/1oz coconut sugar (coconut nectar)
- Pinch of salt
- 1 tbsp coconut oil
- ½ tsp pure vanilla extract

Method

1 Add the chocolate chips, coconut milk, coconut sugar, salt, and coconut oil into your slow cooker. Combine everything together, cover and cook on Low for 2 hours. Do not stir during cooking.

2 After 2 hours, switch off the slow cooker. Add the vanilla, still without stirring. Leave to cool to room temperature, then stir vigorously for a minute or two.

3 Lightly oil a large dish or baking tray. Pour the fudge into pan, cover and refrigerate for 4 hours or until firm.

CHEFS NOTE

Although there is no gluten in chocolate chips, the manufacturing process sometimes makes them unsafe for those with non gluten diets so take care to buy a product labelled as gluten free.

RICE PUDDING

SERVES 4

320
calories per serving

Ingredients

- 150g/5oz long grain pudding rice
- 1 tsp ground cinnamon
- 50g/2oz coconut sugar (coconut nectar)
- 380ml/1½ cups light coconut milk
- 380ml1½ cups semi-skimmed milk
- 100g/3½oz raisins
- 1 tsp pure vanilla extract

Method

1 Add the rice, cinnamon and sugar to your slow cooker and combine well. Stir in the milk and coconut milk, cover and cook on Low for 3-4 hours or until the rice is tender.

2 Stir in the vanilla extract and raisins, and re-cover. Switch off the slow cooker and leave the pudding to set for 10-20 minutes.

3 Serve with extra cinnamon and raisins if you wish.

CHEFS NOTE
Since slow cookers tend to vary, check the consistency of your pudding after 3 hours and see if it needs any longer. Feel free to add more milk if required.

BANANAS AND RUM

130
calories per serving

Ingredients

- 1 tbsp coconut oil
- 3 tbsp honey
- 1 tbsp lemon juice

- ¼ tsp ground cinnamon
- 6 medium bananas, peeled & sliced
- Splash of rum

Method

1 Combine the coconut oil, honey, lemon juice and cinnamon in the slow cooker.

2 Add the banana slices, and toss gently to coat with the honey mixture.

3 Cover and cook on low for 1½ - 2 hours. Stir in a splash of rum, and serve.

CHEFS NOTE
Canola oil is fine to use rather than coconut oil.

CRISPY SPICED APPLES

220 calories per serving

Ingredients

- 3 eating apples, peeled, cored & diced
- 1 tbsp lemon juice
- 100g/3½oz coconut sugar (coconut nectar)
- 50g/2oz gluten free flour
- 25g/1oz gluten free oats
- 1 tsp ground cinnamon
- ½ tsp ground nutmeg
- ¼ tsp all spice
- Salt to taste
- 2 tbsp butter

Method

1 Spread the apples in your bottom of the slow cooker. Add the lemon juice and combine so that the apples are coated. Stir in half the sugar and the cinnamon.

2 In a small bowl, mix the flour, oats, the remaining sugar, nutmeg, all spice, and salt. Use your fingers and thumbs to rub the butter into the mixture until you create a consistency of crumbs.

3 Sprinkle the crumb mixture over the apples. Cover and cook on Low for 4 hours or until the apples are tender.

CHEFS NOTE

Oats contain no gluten, but they can become contaminated by proximity to wheat, so if you need to be careful, buy oats labelled as gluten free.

SPICED APPLES WITH CREAM

135
calories per
serving

Ingredients

- 4 eating apples, peeled, cored and sliced
- 2 tbsp honey
- ½ tsp ground cinnamon
- ½ tsp ground cloves
- 25g/1oz butter, sliced
- 1 tbsp low-fat whipped cream or crème fraiche

Method

Tip the apples into the slow cooker and toss them with the honey, cinnamon, cloves, and butter.

Cover and cook on Low for 4-5 hours, or until the apples are very tender.

Serve with a spoonful of cream.

CHEFS NOTE
Be careful not to overcook your apples or they'll turn into apple sauce!

TAPIOCA PUDDING

324 calories per serving

Ingredients

- 2 eggs
- 1lt/4 cups skimmed milk
- 150g/5oz brown sugar
- 75g/3oz pearl tapioca
- 1 tsp vanilla extract

Method

1 Use a fork to beat the eggs in a cup.

2 Add all the ingredients to the slow cooker and mix well. Cover and cook on Low for 5-6 hours, stirring occasionally.

3 Serve warm.

CHEFS NOTE
Use tapioca pearls rather than powder if possible

OATS AND MAPLE SYRUP

357 calories per serving

Ingredients

- 360ml/1½ cups skimmed milk
- 360ml/1½ cups water
- Cooking spray
- 2 apples, peeled, cored & cubed
- 100g/3½oz gluten free oats
- 2 tbsp brown sugar
- 1½ tsp butter, softened
- ¼ tsp ground cinnamon
- ¼ tsp salt
- 60ml/¼ cup maple syrup
- 2 tbsp hazelnuts, chopped

Method

1 Pour the milk and water into a pan and bring to the boil, stirring frequently.

2 Coat the slow cooker with cooking spray to prevent sticking. Pour in the hot milk mixture. Add the cubed apples, oats, sugar, butter, cinnamon and salt. Stir well. Cover and cook on Low for 7 hours or until the oats are tender.

3 Spoon into bowls, top with maple syrup and chopped hazelnuts.

CHEFS NOTE
Also good served with ice cream.

TROPICAL TAPIOCA

212 calories per serving

Ingredients

- Cooking spray
- 175g/6oz sugar
- 75g/3oz pearl tapioca
- 2 x 400ml/14oz tins light coconut milk
- 1 large egg
- 100g/3½oz fresh pineapple, finely chopped
- 40g/1½oz coconut flakes

Method

1 Coat the slow cooker with cooking spray to prevent sticking. Add the sugar, tapioca & coconut milk and whisk together. Cover and cook on Low for 2 hours or until the tapioca is transparent.

2 Crack the egg into a bowl, beat with a fork and stir the egg mixture into the tapioca in the slow cooker.

3 Cover and cook on Low for 30 minutes. Switch off the slow cooker. Stir the pineapple into the tapioca mixture. Cover once more and leave to stand for 30 minutes. Serve either warm or chilled. Top each serving with the coconut flakes.

CHEFS NOTE
Tinned pineapple also works fine for this recipe.

SPICED APPLE CAKE

238 calories per serving

Ingredients

- Cooking spray
- 100g/3½oz all-purpose gluten free flour
- 25g/1oz dark brown sugar
- ½ tsp baking soda
- 1 tsp ground cinnamon
- ¼ tsp baking powder
- Pinch salt
- Pinch ground nutmeg
- Pinch ground cloves

- 125g/4oz unsweetened apple sauce
- 60ml/¼ cup low-fat buttermilk
- 25g/1oz butter, melted
- ½ tbsp vanilla extract
- 1 small egg
- 100g/3½oz dried apple slices, coarsely chopped
- ½ tsp icing sugar (optional)

Method

1 Coat the slow cooker with cooking spray. Line the bottom with parchment paper, lengthwise and breadthwise. Coat the parchment with cooking spray too.

2 Combine the flour, brown sugar, baking soda, cinnamon, baking powder, salt, nutmeg and cloves in a bowl. In another bowl, combine together the apple sauce, buttermilk, butter, vanilla and egg to create a sauce. Stir this sauce mixture into the flour mixture until it's smooth. Add the dried apple and combine.

3 Place the contents of the bowl into the slow cooker, spreading it into an even layer. Cover and cook on High for 1 - 1½ hours or until the cake has risen.

4 Remove the cake. Cut it into wedges and sprinkle with icing sugar.

CHEFS NOTE
A blend of gluten free flours works best in baking. You can buy these blends in most supermarkets.

ALMOND AND RASPBERRY CHEESECAKE

390 calories per serving

Ingredients

- 16 amoretti biscuits, broken into crumbs
- 2 tbsp butter, melted
- 1 tbsp sugar
- Cooking spray
- 450g/1lb fat-free cream cheese, softened and divided
- 225g/8oz reduced fat cream cheese, softened
- 150g/5oz brown sugar
- 1 tbsp gluten free flour
- 2 large eggs
- ¾ tsp almond extract
- A handful of fresh raspberries

Method

1 For the crust, combine the biscuit crumbs, butter and sugar with a fork until moist. Gently press the mixture into the bottom of a 7-inch baking dish coated with cooking spray.

2 For the filling, blend together the fat free and fat-reduced cheeses. Add the sugar and flour and beat well. Add the eggs, 1 at a time, beating well after each. Stir in the almond extract. Pour the cheese mixture over the crust in the baking dish.

3 Pour the hot water into your slow cooker. Place a rack inside that is higher than the water level. Place the dish with the cheesecake on the rack, and cover with several layers of paper towels.

4 Replace the lid on the slow cooker and cook on High for 2 hours or until the middle of the cheesecake sets (it should barely move when the dish is touched). Uncover the slow cooker. Switch it off and run a knife around outside edge of the baking dish. Leave the cheesecake standing in the slow cooker for an hour and then remove it.

5 Cool to room temperature. Cover and chill in the fridge for at least 6 hours. Cut into wedges, and top with a few raspberries.

CHEFS NOTE

Traditional Amoretti biscuits are made with almonds and should therefore be gluten free, but check the label to be sure!

88

VANILLA CUSTARD

195
calories per serving

Ingredients

- 2 x 170g tins evaporated low-fat milk
- 120ml/½ cup skimmed milk
- 1 tsp vanilla paste
- 1 large egg, lightly beaten
- 2 large egg yolks
- 75g/3oz sugar

Method

1 Pour both kinds of milk into a saucepan. Bring to a simmer, then remove the pan from the heat and add the vanilla paste. Whisk until blended.

2 In a bowl, whisk the egg, egg yolks and sugar. Gradually add the hot milk, beating vigorously with a whisk. Pour the egg mixture through a sieve into a bowl.

3 Place 4 metal canning jar bands in the bottom of your slow cooker. Ladle the egg mixture evenly into 4 ramekins. Cover the ramekins with foil. Set 1 ramekin on each band, making sure ramekins do not touch each other or the sides of slow cooker. Pour hot water into the slow cooker to a depth of 1 inch up the sides of the ramekins.

4 Cover and cook on High for 1¾ hours, or until the custard is 'set'. Remove the ramekins from the slow cooker, and cool on a wire rack.

5 Serve warm or chilled.

CHEFS NOTE
Using evaporated milk should prevent the custard from curdling.

Other COOKNATION TITLES

If you enjoyed **The Skinny Gluten Free Slow Cooker Recipe Book** you may also be interested in other cookbooks in the CookNation series.

You can browse all titles at **www.bellmackenzie.com**

Thank you.

Printed in Great Britain
by Amazon